HASHIMOTO'S DIET COOKBOOK FOR BEGINNERS

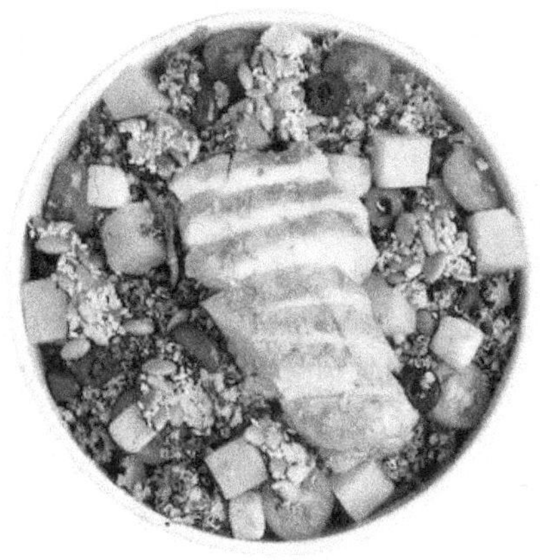

"Delicious and Wholesome Meals for Hashimoto's Warriors"

Allie Nagel

Copyright © 2023 by Allie Nagel

DISCLAIMER

This cookbook is intended to provide general information and recipes. The recipes provided in this cookbook are not intended to replace or be a substitute for medical advice from a physician.

The reader should consult a healthcare professional for any specific medical advice, diagnosis or treatment.

Any specific dietary advice provided in this cookbook is not intended to replace or be a substitute for medical advice from a physician.

The author is not responsible or liable for any adverse effects experienced by readers of this cookbook as a result of following the recipes or dietary advice provided.

The author makes no representations or warranties of any kind (express or implied) as to the accuracy, completeness, reliability or suitability of the recipes provided in this cookbook.

The author disclaims any and all liability for any damages arising out of the use or misuse of the recipes provided in this cookbook.

The reader must also take care to ensure that the recipes provided in this cookbook are prepared and cooked safely. The recipes provided in this cookbook are for informational purposes only and should not be used as a substitute for professional medical advice, diagnosis or treatment.

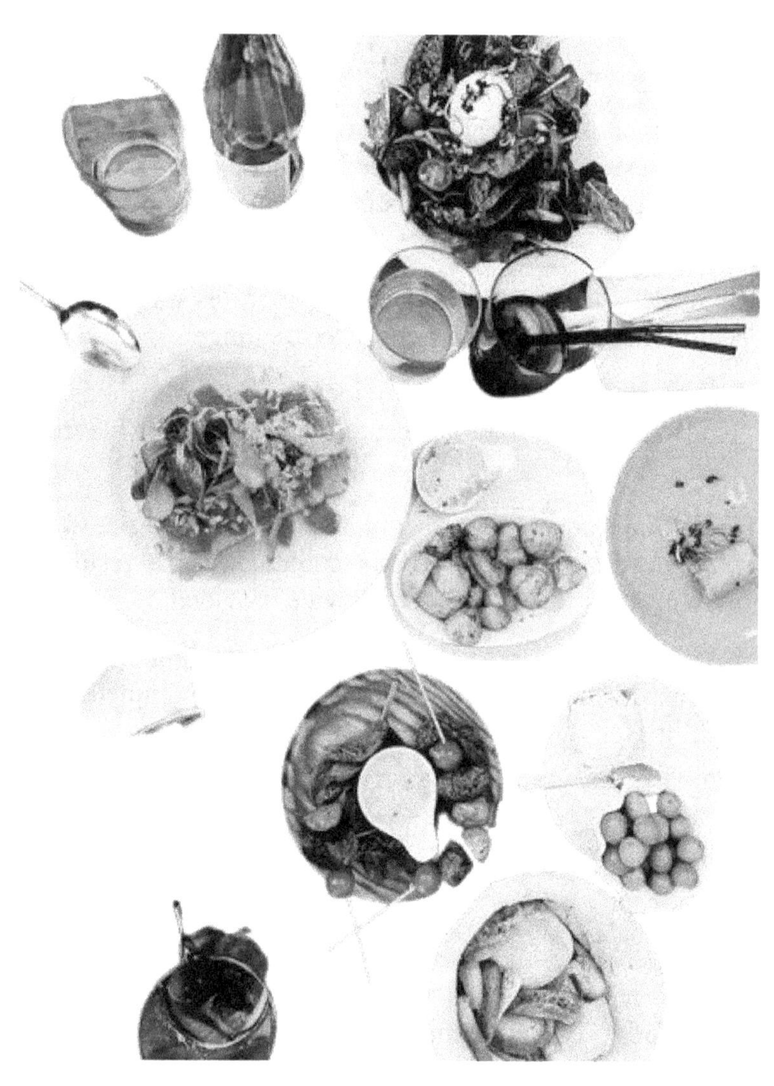

TABLE OF CONTENTS

INTRODUCTION

Mrs. Tina was a kindhearted soul with dreams as big as the sky.

However, fate had dealt her a cruel hand in the form of Hashimoto's disease.

This chronic condition, an autoimmune disorder affecting the thyroid gland, cast a shadow over every aspect of his life.

Tina was no stranger to the debilitating effects of Hashimoto's. Fatigue engulfed him like a neverending fog, stealing away his energy and vitality.

 Her once vibrant spirit was crushed beneath the weight of constant exhaustion. Simple tasks became monumental challenges, leaving him feeling defeated and helpless.

Not only did the physical toll of Hashimoto's affect her, but it also took a toll on her mental and emotional wellbeing.

Depression and anxiety became unwelcome companions, as the relentless symptoms of the disease tested her resilience. Tina felt trapped, as if her body had turned against her, robbing her of the life she so desperately desired.

But in the depths of despair, a glimmer of hope emerged. Tina embarked on a journey of selfdiscovery and empowerment.

She began researching the effects of diet and lifestyle on autoimmune diseases and discovered a wealth of knowledge and testimonies from others who had successfully managed their Hashimoto's through simple changes.

Armed with this newfound information, Tina transformed his life.

She bid farewell to processed foods laden with chemicals and embraced a wholesome, nutrientrich diet. Fresh fruits, vegetables, lean proteins, and whole grains became his allies in the battle against his condition.

Gradually, her strength and stamina returned, and with them came a renewed sense of purpose.

Over time, Tina's dedication paid off. Her energy levels soared, and the fog of fatigue lifted. Her mood improved and the shackles of depression and anxiety loosened their grip. She felt alive again, ready to conquer the world.

CHAPTER 1

An Overview of Hashimotos Disease

Hashimoto's disease is the most common cause of hypothyroidism, a condition in which the thyroid gland does not produce enough thyroid hormones to meet the body's needs.

In Hashimoto's disease, the immune system mistakenly identifies the thyroid gland as a threat and begins to attack it. This immune response leads to inflammation and damage to the thyroid tissue over time.

As a result, the thyroid gland becomes unable to produce sufficient amounts of thyroid hormones, including thyroxine (T4) and triiodothyronine (T3).

The exact cause of Hashimoto's disease is not fully understood, but it is believed to involve a combination of genetic predisposition and environmental triggers.

Women are more commonly affected than men, and the condition often develops during middle age, although it can occur at any age.

One of the challenges in diagnosing Hashimoto's disease is that it can progress slowly and its symptoms can be subtle or mimic those of other conditions.

Some common symptoms include fatigue, weight gain, constipation, sensitivity to cold, dry skin, hair loss, muscle weakness, depression, and memory problems.

In some cases, individuals may also experience a goiter, which is an enlargement of the thyroid gland.

Diagnosis of Hashimoto's disease involves a combination of medical history, physical examination, and blood tests to measure levels of thyroid hormones (T4 and T3) and thyroidstimulating hormone (TSH).

Additionally, the presence of specific antibodies, such as thyroid peroxidase antibodies (TPOAb) and thyroglobulin antibodies (TgAb), can help confirm the autoimmune nature of the disease.

While Hashimoto's disease cannot be cured, it can be effectively managed with lifelong treatment.

The mainstay of treatment is hormone replacement therapy, which involves taking synthetic thyroid hormones (levothyroxine) to restore normal hormone levels in the body.

Regular monitoring of thyroid hormone levels through blood tests is essential to ensure the appropriate dosage of medication.

In addition to medication, lifestyle modifications can also play a role in managing Hashimoto's disease. These may include adopting a healthy diet, exercising regularly, managing stress levels, getting enough sleep, and avoiding tobacco smoke and excessive alcohol consumption.

10 Benefits of Hashimotos Diet

1.Reduced inflammation: A Hashimoto's diet focuses on antiinflammatory foods, which can help reduce inflammation in the body. This can alleviate symptoms such as joint pain, fatigue, and brain fog.

2. Support for thyroid function: A wellbalanced diet can provide essential nutrients that support thyroid function. Consuming foods rich in iodine, selenium, and zinc may be beneficial for thyroid health.

3. Improved energy levels: A diet tailored for Hashimoto's can help stabilize blood sugar levels and provide a steady source of energy. This can prevent energy crashes and alleviate fatigue.

4. Weight management: Hashimoto's disease is often associated with weight gain or difficulty losing weight. A Hashimoto's diet emphasizes nutrientdense foods and portion control, which can support healthy weight management.

5. Gut health optimization: A Hashimoto's diet promotes gut health by including probioticrich foods, fiber, and avoiding triggers like gluten and processed foods.

6. Enhanced nutrient absorption: People with Hashimoto's may have impaired nutrient absorption due to gut issues. A diet rich in whole, unprocessed foods can optimize nutrient absorption and ensure the body receives adequate vitamins and minerals.

7. Balancing blood sugar levels: Hashimoto's patients may be more prone to blood sugar imbalances. A diet that limits refined sugars and focuses on complex carbohydrates, fiber, and healthy fats can help stabilize blood sugar levels.

8. Reduced food sensitivities: Some individuals with Hashimoto's may have underlying food sensitivities that exacerbate their symptoms. Following an elimination diet or identifying trigger foods can help reduce inflammation and improve overall wellbeing.

9. Enhanced immune function: A Hashimoto's diet emphasizes immuneboosting foods such as fruits, vegetables, and omega3 fatty acids. This can support a stronger immune system, reducing the risk of infections and supporting overall health.

10. Psychological wellbeing: Eating a nutrientrich diet and managing symptoms effectively can have positive effects on mental health. Improved energy levels, reduced brain fog, and a sense of control over one's health can contribute to a better overall mood and wellbeing.

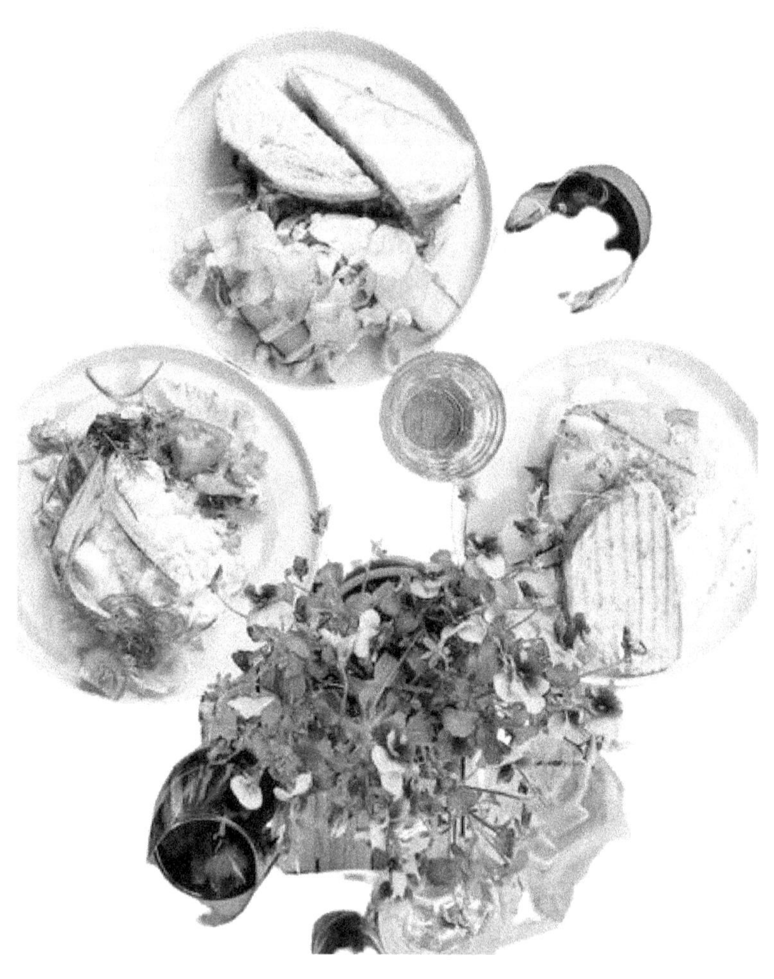

CHAPTER 2

Meal Plan

DAY 1

Breakfast: Seeded Crusted Cod served with Spinach

Lunch: Cucumber and Avocado Salad

Dinner: Coconut Curry with Turmeric

DAY 2

Breakfast: Coconut and Almond Flour Pancakes

Lunch: Lentil and Chicken Soup

Dinner: Salmon with Avocado Salsa

DAY 3

Breakfast: Vegetable Omelette with Coconut Oil

Lunch: Kale, Apples, and Hazelnut Salad

Dinner: Quinoa Buddha Bowls with Broccoli and Mushrooms

DAY 4

Breakfast: Apple and Almond Butter Porridge

Lunch: Salmon and veggies salad

Dinner: Curried Lentils with Spinach

DAY 5

Breakfast: Spicy Brown Rice Breakfast Bowl

Lunch: Quinoa Bowl

Dinner: Butternut Squash and Mushroom Stirfry

DAY 6

Breakfast: AsianStyle Salmon and Kale Bowl

Lunch: Roasted Turkey and Spinach Fajitas

Dinner: Roasted Arugula with Walnuts and Turmeric

DAY 7

Breakfast: Banana and Blueberry Chia Seed Pudding

Lunch: Roasted Carrot and Arugula Salad

Dinner: Lentil and Vegetable Stew

DAY 8

Breakfast: Broccoli Frittata

Lunch: Chicken, Avocado, and Brown Rice Bowl

Dinner: Salmon with Asparagus

DAY 9

Breakfast: Avocado Egg Toast

Lunch: Grilled Shrimp and Broccoli with Herbs

Dinner: Apple and Spinach Salad

DAY 10

Breakfast: Coconut and Pumpkin Seed Granola

Lunch: Grilled Turkey Burger with Quinoa

Dinner: Zucchini noodles

DAY 11

Breakfast: Seeded Crusted Cod served with Spinach

Lunch: Cucumber and Avocado Salad

Dinner: Coconut Curry with Turmeric

DAY 12

Breakfast: Coconut and Almond Flour Pancakes

Lunch: Lentil and Chicken Soup

Dinner: Salmon with Avocado Salsa

DAY 13

Breakfast: Vegetable Omelette with Coconut Oil

Lunch: Kale, Apples, and Hazelnut Salad

Dinner: Quinoa Buddha Bowls with Broccoli and Mushrooms

DAY 14

Breakfast: Apple and Almond Butter Porridge

Lunch: Salmon and veggies salad

Dinner: Curried Lentils with Spinach

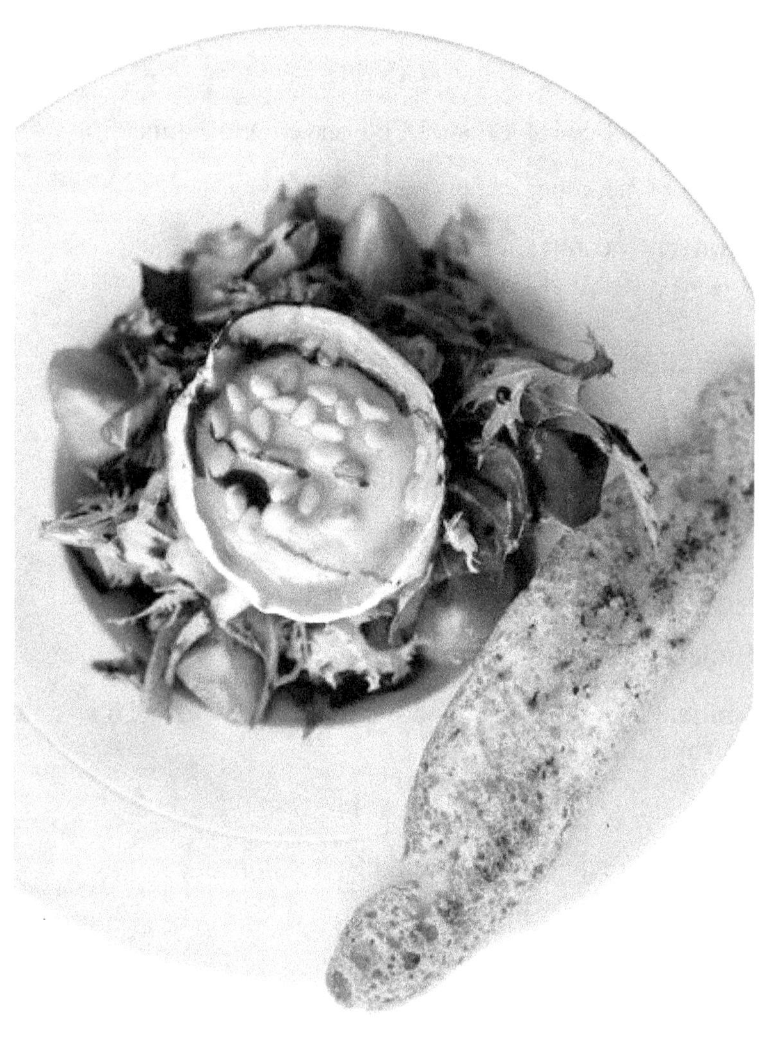

CHAPTER 3

BREAKFAST

Seeded Crusted Cod served with Spinach

Preparing this nutrientrich and omega3rich cod dish is an excellent way to benefit those with Hashimoto's disease. Rich in iron, vitaminA, and other minerals, this dish can help boost your body's defense system.

Ingredients:

4 (4 ounces each) cod fillets

2 teaspoons Dijon mustard

2 teaspoons olive oil

1 teaspoon garlic powder

1/4 cup sesame seeds

2 tablespoons avocado oil

Salt and pepper to taste

2 large handfuls fresh spinach

Preparation Time: 30 minutes

Serving Suggestion: Serve with jasmine rice or sea vegetables

Method of Preparation:

1. Preheat oven to 425°F and line a baking sheet with parchment paper.

2. In a shallow bowl, combine Dijon mustard, olive oil, garlic powder, sesame seeds, salt and pepper.

3. Dip each cod fillet in the mustard mixture and coat both sides with the seed mixture. Place on the prepared baking sheet.

4. Brush each fillet with avocado oil.

5. Bake for 10 minutes or until the edges of the fish are golden brown.

6. Heat a large skillet over mediumhigh heat and add spinach. Saute for 3 minutes or until just wilted.

Coconut and Almond Flour Pancakes Vegetable

Enjoy a light and nutritious start to your day with this delightful combination of coconut and almond flour pancakes.

It is high in fiber and can be beneficial for someone with Hashimoto's disease due to its healthy fats and low sugar content.

Ingredients:

¾ cup almond flour

¼ cup coconut flour

½ teaspoon baking soda

¼ teaspoon salt

2 tablespoons coconut oil, melted

2 tablespoons honey

1 teaspoon vanilla extract

2 eggs

2 tablespoons wild blueberries

2 tablespoons coconut flakes

Preparation Time: 20 minutes

Serving Suggestion: Serve with sliced bananas and almond butter

Method of Preparation:

1. In a large bowl, combine almond flour, coconut flour, baking soda, and salt.

2. In a separate bowl, mix together melted coconut oil, honey, and vanilla extract.

3. Beat eggs and add to the coconut oil mixture.

4. Add the wet ingredients to the dry ingredients and mix until combined.

5. Add wild blueberries and coconut flakes and mix.

6. Heat a nonstick skillet over medium heat.

7. Add about ¼ cup batter for each pancake.

8. Cook for 23 minutes or until bubbles form in the center of the pancake and the edges become firm.

9. Flip and cook for an additional 2 minutes or until both sides are golden brown.

Omelette with Coconut Oil

An omelette made with coconut oil is an excellent way to get all of the health benefits of coconut oil but in an easy and delicious way. Beneficial for those with Hashimoto's disease, it is packed with protein and healthy fats.

Ingredients:

2 eggs

2 tablespoons fullfat canned coconut milk

Salt and pepper to taste

2 tablespoons coconut oil

½ cup shredded cooked pork

¼ cup diced red pepper

¼ cup diced onion

Preparation Time: 15 minutes

Serving Suggestion: Serve with a side of avocado slices and a green salad

Method of Preparation:

1. Beat eggs and coconut milk in a medium bowl. Season with salt and pepper to taste.

2. Heat a nonstick skillet over mediumhigh heat.

3. Add coconut oil to the skillet and spread it evenly on the bottom of the skillet.

4. Pour the egg mixture into the skillet and swirl to evenly distribute the eggs.

5. Drop the diced vegetables and pork over the eggs in the skillet.

6. Cook for 57 minutes or until the edges are golden and the center is firm.

7. Carefully flip the omelette and cook for a additional 13 minutes or until the eggs are cooked through.

Apple and Almond Butter Porridge

Start your day off right with this nutritious porridge full of healthy fats and vitamins; perfect for those suffering from Hashimoto's disease!

Ingredients:

2 cups gluten free oats

4 cups water

2 tablespoons cinnamon

1 apple, diced

2 tablespoons almond butter

2 tablespoons honey

Preparation Time: 15 minutes

Serving Suggestion: Serve with chia seeds and chopped walnuts

Method of Preparation:

1. In a large pot, bring water to a boil.

2. Add oats, cinnamon, and diced apple, stirring to combine.

3. Reduce heat to low and simmer for 57 minutes or until oats have softened.

4. Remove from heat and stir in almond butter and honey until combined.

Spicy Brown Rice Breakfast Bowl

Give your morning an added kick of flavor with this protein-packed brown rice breakfast bowl, full of all the essential nutrients needed for those with Hashimoto's disease.

Ingredients:

2 cups cooked brown rice

2 tablespoons coconut oil

1 teaspoon garlic powder

1 teaspoon cumin

1 teaspoon chili powder

2 teaspoons turmeric

½ cup cooked black beans

2 tablespoons diced red onion

1 medium avocado, diced

2 tablespoons cilantro, chopped

1 lime, cut into wedges

Preparation Time: 10 minutes

Serving Suggestion: Serve with cashew cream and diced tomatoes

Method of Preparation:

1. Heat the coconut oil in a large skillet over mediumhigh heat.

2. Add the garlic powder, cumin, chili powder, and turmeric and cook for 1 minute, stirring frequently.

3. Add the cooked rice, black beans, and diced onion and cook for 35 minutes, stirring occasionally.

4. Remove from heat and let cool for a few minutes.

5. Add the diced avocado and chopped cilantro and stir to combine.

AsianStyle Salmon and Kale Bowl

Enjoy a wholesome Asian inspired meal with this salmon and kale bowl, packed with Omega3 fatty acids and antioxidants to nourish those with Hashimoto's disease.

Ingredients:

1 pound salmon, cut into 4 equal pieces

2 tablespoons coconut oil

1 tablespoon sesame oil

2 tablespoons tamari sauce

2 cloves garlic, minced

2 cups kale, finely chopped

2 tablespoons sesame seeds

Preparation Time: 20 minutes

Serving Suggestion: Serve with quinoa and fresh ginger

Method of Preparation:

1. Preheat oven to 400°F and line a baking sheet with parchment paper.

2. Place salmon pieces on the parchment paper and rub with coconut oil.

3. In a small bowl, combine sesame oil, tamari sauce, and garlic.

4. Drizzle the mixture over the salmon pieces.

5. Bake in the preheated oven for 12-15 minutes or until the salmon is cooked through.

6. Heat a nonstick skillet over medium heat.

7. Add the kale and sesame seeds and cook for three minutes or until the kale is wilted.

Banana and Blueberry Chia Seed Pudding

Reap the benefits of chia seeds with this creamy banana and blueberry pudding recipe; rich in fiber and protein it's the perfect meal for those with Hashimoto's.

Ingredients:

1 ½ cups fullfat canned coconut milk

¼ cup chia seeds

2 tablespoons honey

1 teaspoon vanilla extract

½ banana, mashed

½ cup fresh blueberries

Preparation Time: 7 minutes + overnight resting time

Serving Suggestion: Serve with hemp seeds and coconut flakes

Method of Preparation:

1. In a medium bowl, whisk together coconut milk, chia seeds, honey, and vanilla extract until combined.

2. Add mashed banana and whisk to combine.

3. Cover the bowl with plastic wrap and let sit overnight in the refrigerator.

4. The next morning, stir in fresh blueberries.

Broccoli Frittata

Get a hearty dose of fiber and protein from this savory vegetable's frittata; perfect for those with Hashimoto's to get their daily nutrient intake.

Ingredients:

8 eggs

1 head of broccoli

2 tablespoons ghee

1 tablespoon coconut oil

Salt and pepper to taste

Preparation Time: 20 minutes

Serving Suggestion: Serve with a green salad and diced tomatoes

Method of Preparation:

1. Preheat oven to 400°F and grease a 9x13 inch baking dish with ghee.

2. Wash and cut the broccoli into small florets.

3. Heat a nonstick skillet over medium heat.

4. Add coconut oil and broccoli and cook for 57 minutes or until the broccoli is tender.

5. In a medium bowl, whisk eggs and season with salt and pepper.

6. Add the cooked broccoli to the baking dish and pour the egg mixture over the top.

7. Bake in preheated oven for 15-20 minutes or until the eggs are cooked through.

Avocado Egg Toast

Get a double dose of healthy fats and proteins with this avocado and egg toast recipe; ideal for those with Hashimoto's.

Ingredients:

2 slices gluten free bread

1 large avocado, mashed

1 tablespoon olive oil

2 large eggs

Salt and pepper to taste

Preparation Time: 10 minutes

Serving Suggestion: Serve with a sprinkle of chili flakes and cherry tomatoes

Method of Preparation:

1. Spread the mashed avocado on the two slices of bread.

2. Heat a nonstick skillet over medium heat.

3. Add olive oil to the skillet.

4. Crack eggs into the skillet and season with salt and pepper.

5. Cook until the eggs are cooked to your desired doneness.

6. Place the cooked eggs on top of the avocado toast and serve warm with desired accompaniments.

Coconut and Pumpkin Seed Granola

Start your day on a high note with this nutritious granola full of healthy fats, vitamins, and minerals. Perfect for those with Hashimoto's!

Ingredients:

3 cups gluten free rolled oats

½ cup pumpkin seeds

½ cup shredded coconut

¼ cup coconut oil, melted

¼ cup honey

2 teaspoons cinnamon

Pinch of salt

Preparation Time: 20 minutes

Serving Suggestion: Serve with almond milk and fresh fruit

Method of Preparation:

1. Preheat oven to 350°F and line a baking sheet with parchment paper.

2. In a medium bowl, combine oats, pumpkin seeds, and shredded coconut.

3. In a small bowl, whisk together melted coconut oil, honey, cinnamon, and salt.

4. Pour the wet ingredients over the dry ingredients and stir until evenly combined.

5. Spread the mixture evenly on the prepared baking sheet.

6. Bake for 10 minutes or until golden brown.

7. Let cool and serve with desired accompaniments.

LUNCH

Cucumber and Avocado Salad

Fill your plate with this light and healthy cucumber and avocado salad, full of nutrition and vitamins necessary for a

Hashimoto's management diet and offering a delicious and crunchy break from the everyday.

Ingredients:

1 cucumber, sliced

2 avocados, diced

2 tablespoons freshly squeezed lemon juice

2 tablespoons olive oil

1 teaspoon salt

1 teaspoon freshly ground black pepper

Preparation Time: 15 min

Method of Preparation:

1. Slice the cucumber and dice the avocado.

2. In a small bowl, whisk together the lemon juice, olive oil, salt and black pepper to make the dressing.

3. In a large bowl, combine the cucumber and avocado.

4. Drizzle the dressing over the salad and toss until everything is evenly coated.

Serving Suggestion: Serve with grilled chicken or fish for a healthy and delicious meal.

Lentil and Chicken Soup

Bursts of flavor and nutrients abound with this traditional lentil and chicken soup. Filled with protein and healthy fats to fight inflammation, it makes a nourishing meal for offering relief to those with Hashimoto's disease.

Ingredients:

1 cup dry lentils

1 tablespoon olive oil

1 large onion, chopped

3 cloves garlic, minced

4 cups chicken broth

2 cups cooked shredded chicken

1 teaspoon ground cumin

1 teaspoon smoked paprika

1 teaspoon salt

1/2 teaspoon freshly ground black pepper

Preparation Time: 40 Minutes

Method of Preparation:

1. In a medium saucepan, heat the olive oil over mediumhigh heat.

2. Add the onion and garlic and cook until soft, about 5 minutes.

3. Add the lentils and chicken broth and bring to a boil.

4. Reduce the heat to a simmer and cook for 20 minutes, or until the lentils are tender.

5. Add the cooked chicken, cumin, smoked paprika, salt and pepper and simmer for 5 more minutes.

Serving Suggestion: Serve with crusty bread and a simple green salad for a complete meal.

Kale, Apples, and Hazelnut Salad

Enjoy the wholesomeness and sweetness in this kale, apple, and hazelnut salad. The powerful combination of nutrients provides essential dietary support for Hashimoto's, and even adds a crunch.

Ingredients:

2 cups kale, chopped

1 apple, chopped

1/4 cup hazelnuts, chopped

1/4 cup extravirgin olive oil

2 tablespoons freshly squeezed lemon juice

1/2 teaspoon salt

Preparation Time: 15 Minutes

Method of Preparation:

1. In a large bowl, combine the kale, apple, and hazelnuts.

2. In a small bowl, whisk together the olive oil, lemon juice and salt to make the dressing.

3. Drizzle the dressing over the salad and toss until everything is evenly coated.

Serving Suggestion: Serve as a side dish accompanied by grilled chicken or fish.

Salmon and Veggies Salad

Packed with healthy fats, fresh vegetables, and delicious salmon, this salad is a great choice for those looking to add more omega3s to their Hashimoto's diet. Its plentiful nutritional benefits make it a must have for meal planning.

Ingredients:

1/2-pound cooked salmon, diced

1/2 red bell pepper, diced

1/2 head broccoli, chopped

1 cup cooked quinoa

2 tablespoons extravirgin olive oil

2 tablespoons freshly squeezed lemon juice

1/2 teaspoon salt

Preparation Time: 20 Minutes

Method of Preparation:

1. In a medium bowl, combine the salmon, bell pepper, broccoli and quinoa.

2. In a small bowl, whisk together the olive oil, lemon juice and salt to make the dressing.

3. Drizzle the dressing over the salad and toss until everything is evenly coated.

Serving Suggestion: Serve as a light lunch or dinner accompanied with a side of fruit.

Quinoa Bowl

Promote thyroid health and reduce inflammation with this hearty quinoa bowl. Nutrientdense, vitaminenriched ingredients will fill you up and provide energy throughout the day.

Ingredients:

1 cup cooked quinoa

1/4 cup cooked chickpeas

1/4 cup diced red bell pepper

1 cup cooked spinach

3 tablespoons olive oil

2 tablespoons freshly squeezed lemon juice

1 teaspoon salt

Preparation Time: 10 Minutes

Method of Preparation:

1. In a large bowl, combine the cooked quinoa, chickpeas, bell pepper and spinach.

2. In a small bowl, whisk together the olive oil, lemon juice and salt to make the dressing.

3. Drizzle the dressing over the quinoa bowl and toss until everything is evenly coated.

Serving Suggestion: Serve as a light lunch or dinner alongside a side salad or roasted vegetables.

Roasted Turkey and Spinach Fajitas

This southwest style fajitas dish is a great way to supplement the healthy balance of proteins and fats necessary for managing Hashimoto's disease. Roasted turkey and spinach bring flavors and aromas that will tantalize your taste buds and provide essential nutrition.

Ingredients:

1 pound ground turkey

1 teaspoon chili powder

1 teaspoon cumin

1 teaspoon smoked paprika

1 teaspoon garlic powder

1 teaspoon salt

1/2 teaspoon freshly ground black pepper

1 onion, chopped

1 bell pepper, chopped

1 cup cooked spinach

1 tablespoon extravirgin olive oil

6 wholegrain tortillas

Preparation Time: 30 Minutes

Method of Preparation:

1. Preheat the oven to 375 degrees Fahrenheit.

2. In a large bowl, combine the ground turkey, chili powder, cumin, smoked paprika, garlic powder, salt and pepper.

3. Spread the turkey mixture on a rimmed baking sheet and top with the onion, bell pepper, and spinach. Drizzle the olive oil over the vegetables.

4. Roast in preheated oven for 20 minutes, or until the turkey is cooked through and the vegetables are tender.

5. Divide the turkey and vegetables among the tortillas and roll up. Serve and enjoy.

Serving Suggestion: Serve with a dollop of sour cream or Greek yogurt and a side of guacamole or salsa.

Roasted Carrot and Arugula Salad

Satisfy your appetite and nourish your body with this roasted carrot and arugula salad. The crunchy texture and savory flavors of the roasted carrots provide antioxidant benefits, while the nutrientrich arugula aids in managing Hashimoto's disease.

Ingredients:

4 carrots, chopped

1 tablespoon olive oil

2 cups baby arugula

2 tablespoons freshly squeezed orange juice

1 teaspoon orange zest

1/4 teaspoon salt

Preparation Time: 25 Minutes

Method of Preparation:

1. Preheat the oven to 400 degrees Fahrenheit.

2. In a medium bowl, toss the carrots with the olive oil.

3. Spread the carrots out on a rimmed baking sheet and roast for 20 minutes, or until they are tender and lightly browned.

4. In a large bowl, combine the roasted carrots, arugula, orange juice, orange zest, and salt.

5. Toss until everything is evenly coated.

Serving Suggestion: Serve as a side dish or add grilled chicken or fish for a more substantial meal.

Chicken, Avocado, and Brown Rice Bowl

Supercharge your body with this chicken, avocado, and brown rice bowl. Packed with essential vitamins and minerals needed for managing Hashimoto's disease, each bite is filled with delicious nourishment.

Ingredients:

1 cup cooked brown rice

1 chicken breast, cooked and diced

1 avocado, diced

1 tablespoon extravirgin olive oil

2 tablespoons freshly squeezed lime juice

1 teaspoon chili powder

1/4 teaspoon salt

Preparation Time: 20 Minutes

Method of Preparation:

1. In a large bowl, combine the brown rice, chicken, and avocado.

2. In a small bowl, whisk together the olive oil, lime juice, chili powder and salt to make the dressing.

3. Drizzle the dressing over the bowl and toss until everything is evenly coated.

Serving Suggestion: Serve as a light lunch or dinner. Top with some crumbled feta cheese and a dollop of Greek yogurt for extra flavor.

Grilled Shrimp and Broccoli with Herbs

Delight in the amazing flavors and superior nutrition of this grilled shrimp and broccoli with herbs. The herbs help add a depth of flavor, while the omega3 rich shrimp fights inflammation in those with Hashimoto's disease.

Ingredients:

1 pound shrimp, deveined and peeled

1 head broccoli, cut into florets

2 tablespoons extravirgin olive oil

2 tablespoons freshly squeezed lemon juice

1/2 teaspoon garlic powder

2 tablespoons chopped fresh parsley

1 teaspoon chopped fresh oregano

1/2 teaspoon sea salt

Preparation Time: 15 Minutes

Method of Preparation:

1. Preheat the grill to medium high heat.

2. In a medium bowl, toss the shrimp and broccoli with the olive oil, lemon juice, garlic powder, parsley, oregano and sea salt.

3. Grill the shrimp and broccoli until the shrimp is cooked through and the broccoli is tender, about 1012 minutes.

Serving Suggestion: Serve with cooked quinoa or brown rice for a complete meal.

Grilled Turkey Burger with Quinoa

Enjoy guilt-free indulgence of this grilled turkey burger with quinoa. Filled with vitamins and minerals that support Hashimoto's management while providing a tasty meal, this meal will have you feeling satisfied but light.

Ingredients:

1 pound ground turkey

1/4 cup cooked quinoa

1/4 cup diced onion

1/4 cup diced red bell pepper

1 teaspoon smoked paprika

1 teaspoon garlic powder

1/2 teaspoon salt

1/4 teaspoon freshly ground black pepper

Preparation Time: 30 Minutes

Method of Preparation:

1. Preheat the grill to medium high heat.

2. In a large bowl, combine the ground turkey, quinoa, onion, bell pepper, smoked paprika, garlic powder, salt and pepper.

3. Form into patties and transfer to the grill. Grill for about 5 minutes per side, or until the burgers are cooked through.

Serving Suggestion: Serve with a side of roasted veggies or a simple green salad for a delicious and balanced meal.

DINNER

Coconut Curry with Turmeric

This creamy and flavorful curry dish is packed with rich spices and healthpromoting turmeric.

It provides crucial nutrients for those suffering from Hashimotos disease, including immunityboosting antioxidants and antiinflammatory properties.

Ingredients:

2 tablespoons olive oil

1 red onion, diced

3 garlic cloves, diced

1 tablespoon freshly grated ginger

3 teaspoons curry powder

1 teaspoon turmeric

1 teaspoon cumin

1 red chili pepper, chopped (optional)

1 can light coconut milk

1 can crushed tomatoes

1 cup vegetable stock

1 teaspoon maple syrup

1 tablespoon tamari

1 teaspoon sea salt

1-pound skinless, boneless salmon fillet, cubed

1/2 cup fresh cilantro for garnish

Preparation Time: 25 minutes

Method of Preparation:

1. Heat oil in a large saucepan over medium heat.

2. Add onion, garlic, ginger, curry powder, turmeric, cumin, and chili pepper (if desired). Cook for 5 minutes until fragrant.

3. Add coconut milk, tomatoes, vegetable stock, maple syrup, tamari, and salt. Stir and bring to a gentle boil.

4. Reduce heat to low and let simmer for 10 minutes.

5. Add cubed salmon and cook until cooked through, about 5 minutes.

6. Serve in individual bowls.

7. Garnish with fresh cilantro, if desired.

Serving Suggestions: Serve with steamed jasmine rice or roasted vegetables for a complete meal.

Salmon with Avocado Salsa

This light and delicious dish combines the healthy fats and minerals of salmon and avocado to provide the essential nutrition needed to treat Hashimotos disease.

Ingredients:

2 tablespoons olive oil

2 cloves garlic, minced

1 teaspoon ground cumin

1 teaspoon paprika

1 teaspoon sea salt

1 pound salmon fillet, cut into 4 portions

1 avocado, peeled, pitted and diced

1/2 red onion, diced

1/2 cup cherry tomatoes, halved

2 tablespoons fresh cilantro, minced

Juice of 1/2 lime

Preparation Time: 15 minutes

Method of Preparation:

1. Preheat oven to 375°F. Grease a baking dish with olive oil or cooking spray.

2. In a small bowl, combine garlic, cumin, paprika, and sea salt.

3. Rub the salmon with the spice mixture and place in the prepared baking dish.

4. Bake for 15 minutes until cooked through.

5. In a medium bowl, combine the diced avocado, red onion, cherry tomatoes, cilantro, and lime juice.

Serving Suggestions: Serve with steamed brown or black rice, or quinoa for a complete meal.

Quinoa Buddha Bowls with Broccoli and Mushrooms

This vegan bowl of highfiber quinoa, broccoli, and mushrooms makes a complete meal packed with vitamins and minerals to support healthy thyroid function.

Ingredients:

2 cups quinoa

1 onion, diced

1 teaspoon minced garlic

1 tablespoon olive oil

3 cups broccoli florets

3 cups sliced mushrooms

1/4 teaspoon sea salt

1/2 teaspoon black pepper

1/4 teaspoon red chili flakes

3 tablespoons lowsodium tamari

1/4 cup fresh lemon juice

1/4 cup toasted almonds

Preparation Time: 25 minutes

Method of Preparation:

1. Start by cooking the quinoa according to package instructions. Set aside.

2. In a large skillet, heat olive oil over mediumhigh heat.

3. Add onion and garlic and cook until fragrant, stirring occasionally, about 2 minutes.

4. Add broccoli, mushrooms, salt, pepper, and chili flakes. Cook for 34 minutes until vegetables are tender.

5. Add cooked quinoa, tamari, and lemon juice. Cook for another 3 minutes, stirring occasionally.

Serving Suggestions: Serve with steamed edamame, cooked greens, or your favorite vegetable for a complete meal.

Curried Lentils with Spinach

Rich in fiber and protein, curried lentils and spinach are a nutritious combination that offer a variety of essential vitamins and minerals needed to treat Hashimotos.

Ingredients:

2 tablespoons olive oil

1 onion, diced

1 tablespoon minced garlic

1 tablespoon curry powder

1 teaspoon ground cumin

1/4 teaspoon ground turmeric

1/4 teaspoon black pepper

1 can (15 ounces) cooked lentils, drained and rinsed

1 can (15 ounces) light coconut milk

2 cups vegetable broth

1 teaspoon sea salt

6 cups baby spinach

1/4 cup fresh cilantro, chopped

Preparation Time: 25 minutes

Method of Preparation:

1. Heat oil in a large saucepan over medium heat.

2. Add onion and garlic and cook until fragrant, about 2 minutes.

3. Add curry powder, cumin, turmeric, and pepper, stirring for 30 seconds.

4. Add lentils, coconut milk, vegetable broth, and salt. Bring to a low boil and cook for 10 minutes.

5. Reduce heat to low and let simmer for another 10 minutes.

6. Remove from heat and stir in spinach and cilantro.

Serving Suggestions: Serve with steamed brown or wild rice, or quinoa for a complete meal.

Butternut Squash and Mushroom Stirfry

This savory-sweet stirfry is filled with cancer-fighting compounds and proteins that helps to reduce inflammation associated with Hashimoto's disease. The mushrooms and butternut squash combine to provide a range of vitamins and minerals for optimal health.

Ingredients:

2 tablespoons olive oil

1 onion, diced

1 tablespoon minced ginger

2 cloves garlic, minced

3 cups cubed butternut squash

3 cups sliced mushrooms

1 teaspoon sea salt

1 teaspoon black pepper

1 teaspoon ground coriander

1/4 cup vegetable stock

1 tablespoon tamari

2 tablespoons sesame oil

2 tablespoons toasted sesame seeds

Preparation Time: 25 minutes

Method of Preparation:

1. Heat oil in a large skillet over medium high heat.

2. Add onion and cook until softened, about 3 minutes.

3. Add ginger and garlic and cook for 1 minute.

4. Add butternut squash and mushrooms and season with salt, pepper, and coriander.

5. Add vegetable stock and cover skillet with a lid. Reduce heat to low and let cook for 10 minutes.

6. Add tamari and sesame oil and cook for another 3 minutes, stirring occasionally.

7. Serve in individual bowls and top with toasted sesame seeds.

Serving Suggestions: Serve over steamed quinoa or brown or wild rice for a complete meal.

Roasted Arugula with Walnuts and Turmeric

This healthy medley of arugula, walnuts, and turmeric helps to reduce inflammation and ease symptoms of Hashimotos disease. The antioxidants in the ingredients offer multiple health benefits, while the flavors create a tasty and healthy addition to any meal.

Ingredients:

2 bunches arugula, washed and dried

2 tablespoons olive oil

1/2 teaspoon sea salt

1/2 teaspoon black pepper

1/2 teaspoon ground turmeric

1/4 cup walnuts, toasted and chopped

Preparation Time: 15 minutes

Method of Preparation:

1. Preheat oven to 375°F.

2. Place arugula on a baking sheet and drizzle with olive oil. Sprinkle with salt, pepper, and turmeric.

3. Toast for 5 minutes until wilted.

4. Remove from oven and place in a serving bowl. Top with toasted walnuts.

Serving Suggestions: Serve the roasted arugula as a side dish with grilled meats or fish for a complete meal.

Zucchini Noodles

These lowcarb, nutrientpacked noodles provide the vitamins and minerals needed to reduce inflammation and improve thyroid function for those suffering from Hashimotos. The freshness of zucchini makes for a delicious and satisfying meal.

Ingredients:

2 tablespoons olive oil

3 large zucchinis, spiralized

1 teaspoon garlic, minced

1/2 teaspoon lemon zest

3 tablespoons freshly squeezed lemon juice

1/4 teaspoon sea salt

1/4 teaspoon black pepper

1/4 cup slivered almonds, toasted

1/4 cup fresh parsley, chopped

Preparation Time: 10 minutes

Method of Preparation:

1. Heat olive oil in a large skillet over mediumhigh heat.

2. Add zucchini noodles and cook for 34 minutes until just wilted.

3. Add garlic, lemon zest, lemon juice, salt, and pepper. Cook for 2 minutes until heated through.

4. Remove from heat and top with toasted almonds and chopped parsley.

Serving Suggestions: Serve the zucchini noodles as a side dish with baked or grilled chicken or fish for a complete meal.

Lentil and Vegetable Stew

This hearty stew provides all the essential vitamins and minerals to manage Hashimotos, as well as reducing inflammation. The combination of proteinfilled lentils and fresh vegetables creates a flavorful and nutritious dish.

Ingredients:

2 tablespoons olive oil

1 onion, diced

2 cloves garlic, minced

1 tablespoon minced ginger

1 teaspoon curry powder

1 teaspoon turmeric

1 teaspoon sea salt

1/2 teaspoon black pepper

2 cups vegetable broth

1 can (15 ounces) cooked lentils, drained and rinsed

2 carrots, peeled and diced

2 celery stalks, diced

1 zucchini, diced

2 cups chopped kale

1/4 cup freshly squeezed lemon juice

Preparation Time: 25 minutes

Method of Preparation:

1. Heat oil in a large saucepan over medium heat.

2. Add onion, garlic, ginger, curry powder, turmeric, salt, and pepper. Cook for 5 minutes until fragrant.

3. Add vegetable broth, lentils, carrots, celery, and zucchini. Bring to a gentle boil and cook for 10 minutes.

4. Reduce heat to low and add kale. Let cook for another 5 minutes.

5. Stir in lemon juice.

Serving Suggestions: Serve the lentil stew as is or over steamed quinoa, brown or wild rice, or cooked quinoa for a complete meal.

Salmon with Asparagus

This classic combination of healthy fats and minerals from the salmon and antioxidants and vitamins in the asparagus help to reduce inflammation and improve the symptoms of Hashimotos disease.

Ingredients:

2 tablespoons olive oil

4 cloves garlic, minced

1 teaspoon sea salt

1/2 teaspoon black pepper

1 pound salmon fillet

1 lemon, cut into wedges

1 pound asparagus, trimmed

Preparation Time: 15 minutes

Method of Preparation:

1. Preheat oven to 375°F. Grease a baking dish with olive oil or cooking spray.

2. In a small bowl, combine garlic, salt, and pepper.

3. Rub the salmon with the spice mixture and place in the prepared baking dish.

4. Add the lemon wedges to the baking dish.

5. Scatter the asparagus around the salmon.

6. Bake for 12-15 minutes until the salmon is cooked through and the asparagus is tender.

Serving Suggestions: Serve the salmon and asparagus with steamed brown or wild rice for a complete meal.

Apple and Spinach Salad

This wholesome salad provides a variety of essential vitamins and minerals to support the reduction of inflammation associated with Hashimoto's disease. Apples and spinach are also rich in antioxidants, making this perfect for an antioxidantrich meal.

Ingredients:

4 cups baby spinach

1 cup chopped apples

1/4 cup toasted almonds nuts

1/4 cup dried cranberries

1/4 cup freshly squeezed lemon juice

1/4 teaspoon sea salt

1/4 cup olive oil

Preparation Time: 10 minutes

Method of Preparation:

1. Place spinach in a large bowl.

2. Top with chopped apples, toasted almonds, and dried cranberries.

3. In a separate bowl, whisk together lemon juice, salt, and olive oil to make a dressing.

4. Pour the dressing over the salad and toss to combine.

Serving Suggestions: Serve as is as a side dish with grilled chicken or fish for a complete meal.

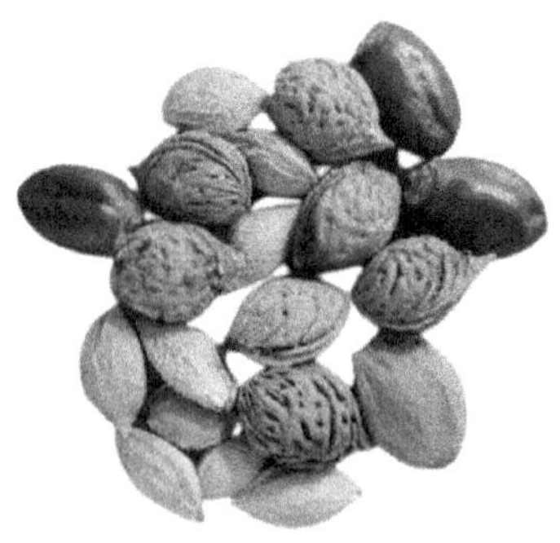

CONCLUSION

In conclusion, Hashimoto's Diet Cookbook for Beginners offers a transformative journey towards health and wellbeing for those living with Hashimoto's disease.

In this culinary exploration, it is important to note that you embarked on a voyage of discovery, uncovering a treasure trove of delectable recipes tailored specifically to support and nourish your body.

More so, this book has given you the opportunity to gain access to a diverse range of recipes but also learned valuable insights into the dietary principles that can positively impact our wellbeing.

Finally, asides recipes and other valuable topics, this book also instills hope and empowers you to take control of your health, one delicious meal at a time.

With this newfound knowledge, I hope you embark on a life long journey of nourishing yourselves and embracing the healing power of food.

Bon appétit!

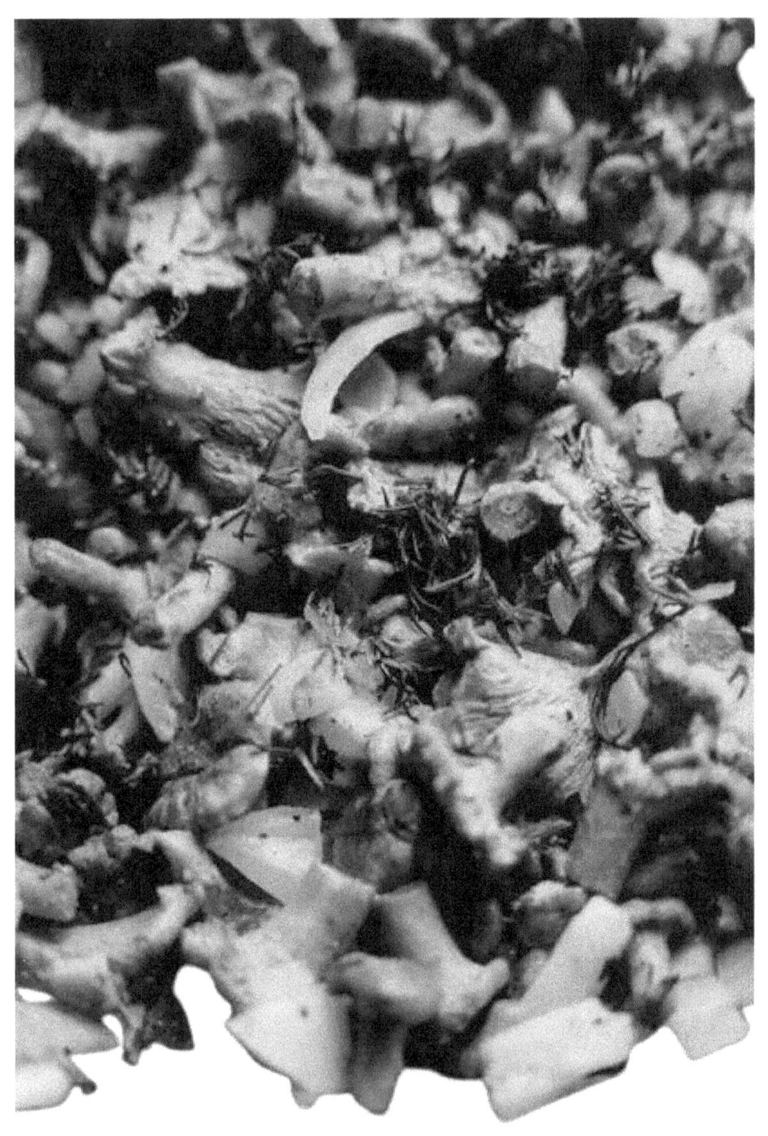